Acid Reflux

I0146515

The First Step In Treating Gastroesophageal Reflux Disease Or Acid Reflux Is Adopting A Healthier Lifestyle

(Manage Acid Reflux And Gerd With Recipes For A Low Acid Diet That Are Actually Delicious)

Anselmo-Rio Huertas

TABLE OF CONTENT

Chapter 1: How Is The Diagnosis Of Acid Reflux Disease Made?

It is time to see your doctor if you experience symptoms of acid reflux more than twice per week or if medications really do not such provide long-term relief. Symptoms such as acid reflux and heartburn are used to diagnose acid reflux disease, particularly if lifestyle changes, antacids, or acid-blocking medications really help alleviate the symptoms.

If these treatments really do not work, or if you are experiencing frequent or severe symptoms, your doctor may order a diagnosis and a search for additional issues. You may require one or more of these tests:

• Barum wallow (esophagram) may indicate ulser or a constriction of the esophagus. You first wallow an oluton to assist with how ur on an X-rau. • Eorhageal manomeeasy try can shesk the function and movement of the eorhagu and lower eorhageal rhnster.

• The doctor inserts a device into your throat and leaves it there for one to two days in order to determine the amount of aspirin in your system.

• Endoscopy can examine your esophagus and stomach for simple problems. The test entails inserting a long, flexible, light-emitting tube containing a saline solution down your throat. The doctor will first numb your throat with an anesthetic and then administer a sedative to make you more comfortable.

• During endosoru, a borumau is taken to examine amrle of tue under a microscope for signs of infection or abnormalities.

Chapter 2 : What Medications Are Available To Treat Acid Reflux?

If over-the-counter antacids and acid blockers really do not alleviate your heartburn, your doctor may prescribe alternative medications, such as:

Presrton-strength acid blotter: Zantac, Tagamet, Pepcid, and Axid can typically relieve heartburn and treat GERD in prescription-strength (typically higher doses).

Proton pump inhibitors are drugs that inhibit acid production more efficiently. Proton rumr inhibitors consist of AsrhexNexumPrevasumPrloes and Protonx.

There are some proton pump inhibitors available without a prescription. Discuss these medications with your health care provider to determine which is best for you.

Chapter 3: A Summary Of Larungorharungoid Reflux

Slent reflux is a condition in which acid from the stomach causes throat discomfort, specifically behind the breastbone in the middle of the body.

It does not aleasy way cause heartburn, but it can cause throat and vocal cord damage.

The condition is also referred to as laryngopharyngeal reflux (LPR).

The stomach's contents include tomahto asad. When these acids easy come into contact with the esophagus and vocal chords, irritation, pain, and easily burning can occur.

These discomforting sensations are caused by acid reflux. A reflux is a backward or reverse flow. In LPR, the contents of the stomach flow back into the esophagus and irritate the throat.

LPR can manifest in infants and adults. It is curable.

If you have ever overindulged in pizza and beer, you may be familiar with acid reflux. Heartburn, vomiting, and diarrhea are all symptoms of reflux.

The symptoms are distinct. However, in some cases, the symptoms of reflux are not so obvious. In quick, they are silent.

Larungorharungeal reflux (LPR) is commonly referred to as silent reflux. LPR doesn't sause anu sumrtoms. The contents of your stomach may reflux into your esophagus, pharynx, and even your nasal passages, and you may not even be aware of it until more serious symptoms appear as a result of stomach acid damage.

Chapter 4: How To Repair The Damage Caused By Acid To The Body

Saliva, urine, and blood are just a few bodily fluids that contribute significantly to how our body functions. On the other hand, an accumulation of too much acid in these fluids can result in serious illnesses and health simple problems. In the following section, you'll learn how to address these simple problems and get started on the path to better health.

What is the meaning of the term "Acidity"?

Acidity or acidosis refers to an increase in the amount of acid that has accumulated in our bodies. For our biological fluids to function properly, a pH of 7.0 or higher is required. All substances with a pH below 7 are considered acidic.

If you suffer from any of the following conditions, you may have an excess of acid in your body:

• Difficulty losing weight • Muscle aches and pains • Fragile bones or osteoporosis • Teeth simple problems • Fatigue or insomnia • An increase in mucus production • Dermatological issues

Numerous factors contribute to an increase in our bodies' acidity. The accumulation of acid in our bodies is influenced not only by the types of food we consume, but also by the beverages we consume. Consuming alcohol and caffeine, as well as processed foods and sugar, raises the acidity levels in the body. In addition to affecting the development of acidosis, the air we breathe and other environmental factors can also have an impact.

Methods for Success

Even though you may believe the damage is irreparable, there is still a chance it can be repaired. Follow these simple guidelines if you really want to easily reduce acid accumulation in your body:

Alkaline water provides the superior hydration your body requires and is one of the easiest easy way to easily reduce acidity in the body. If you maintain a healthy level of hydration, your body will naturally eliminate excess acid from the digestive tract.

Eliminate the Waste — The acid levels in our bodies are influenced by numerous factors, including processed foods, sugary beverages, caffeine, and alcohol. They remove calcium and magnesium from our muscles and bones, making us more prone to developing osteoporosis and other diseases.

Change your Diet – Easily eating well and living a healthy lifestyle go hand in hand, but it is the food you basically consume that can really help neutralize the acid that builds up in your body. Vegetables that appear dark green and leafy, such as kale, broccoli, arugula, and celery, contain alkalizing properties that can neutralize acid. Calcium and magnesium, two minerals lost in the body as a result of acidosis, can be replaced by easily eating dried fruit and seafood.

However, if your kidneys are unable to control an excess of acidity, this can also result in bone and muscle damage. If the internal environment of the body becomes excessively acidic, calcium will be removed from the bones to neutralize the acidity. This can eventually result in bone deterioration, leading to osteoporosis.

Chapter 5: How To Treat Heartburn Without Medication

It is sound advice that prevention is preferable to treatment. This is the reality regarding acid reflux. On a short-term basis, medication may appear to be the simpler option; just PIP one pill and you're done. Doctors and researchers concur, however, that non-medication-related lifestyle changes and improvements are much more durable and effective over the long term. Thus, bearing this in mind. This chapter will discuss some of the few just thing you can really do to easily manage acid reflux without the use of medication.

Easily eating in moderation and slowly.

When the stomach is extremely full, the internal pressure rises. This causes more food to easy try to push back and reflux into the esophagus. k/a grazing. Basically consume balanced small meals. Eat frequently and easily Avoid consuming three large meals per day. You can instead basically consume food five, six, or more times per day. This reduces pressure on the lower esophagus and aids in controlling reflux.

Easily Avoid particular foods

People with acid reflux were once advised to easily Avoid all foods except the most bland ones. However, this is no longer the case. People with reflux can effectively easily manage their symptoms by easily avoiding a handful of very common triggers. These foods are more likely to cause acid reflux. Mint, fatty foods, spicy foods, tomatoes, onions, garlic, coffee, tea, chocolate, and alcohol are among these. If you regularly basically consume any of these foods, you may really want to easy try eliminating them to see if your reflux such improves, and then reintroducing them one by one. Eat only the ones that are safe and discard the rest until you feel better.

Don't drink carbonated beverages

The carbonation of carbonated beverages is caused by the pressurized gas contained within them. When you basically consume these beverages, gas is produced, causing you to burp. Burping causes acid to enter the esophagus and exacerbates reflux. Instead of sparkling water and cold drinks, basically consume flat water.

Stay awake after meals (standing or sitting).

Gravity aids in retaining stomach acid. When a person lies down with a full stomach, food is pushed up into the esophagus, causing reflux. Make it a habit to finish easily eating at least three hours prior to bedtime. Easily Avoid just taking naps after lunch and easily eating late suppers and midnight snacks to easily reduce your risk of acid reflux.

Additionally, vigorous exercise should be avoided for a couple of hours after eating. An after-dinner stroll or casual walk is acceptable, but a strenuous workout, especially one that involves bending over, can cause acid to enter the esophagus.

Sleep on a bed with an incline.

Another way to let Gravity really do its job is by sleeping on an inclined bed. When your bed is inclined, gravity prevents food and liquid from rising into your esophagus, effectively preventing reflux. Ideal head height is 6 to 8 inches higher than foot height. You can accomplish this by placing "extra-tall" bed risers on the bed's legs to support the bed's head. You can also easy try supporting your upper body with a foam wedge. Just make sure you have uniform support and don't interfere with your natural sleep.

Easily reduce weight.

The supporting muscular structure of the lower esophageal sphincter aids in keeping it tight and closed. When a person is overweight, the esophageal sphincter is weakened due to strain on this muscular structure. This is the initial cause of reflux issues.

Obesity is associated with a statistically significant increase in the risk of reflux (GERD) symptoms, erosive esophagitis, sore throat, and esophageal cancer, according to studies. They also discovered that this risk increases proportionally with easily weight gain. It is preferable to eat less, exercise more, and lose weight rather than undergo surgery or take acid reflux medications.

If you smoke, quit.

Nicotine, an essential component of tobacco, is believed to relax the ring of lower esophageal muscles that keep stomach acid in the stomach. Every time you smoke, this ring relaxes, allowing acid to seep up and cause that easily burning sensation. In addition, smoking reduces the amount of mucus your body normally produces. Mucus is necessary to prevent acid from attacking the stomach and esophagus from the inside, so when mucus production decreases, symptoms of reflux worsen.

Additionally, the majority of smokers have chest issues that cause them to cough frequently. Coughing increases abdominal pressure, which in turn increases acid reflux. Every time you cough, acid is expelled upwards and heartburn worsens.

Health-wise, nicotine gums and patches are safer options. They will assist you in kicking your habit and are less likely to cause heartburn. One small study found no increased risk of heartburn among nicotine patch users. The extent to which smoking destroys the human body internally goes without saying.

Chapter 6: Beverages That Prevent Heartburn

Some beverages may not exacerbate acid reflux symptoms, but others may.

In addition to the below-recommended beverages, consider sipping liquids rather than guzzling them. This may really help alleviate acid reflux symptoms. Numerous sips of water can aid the esophagus's ability to flush acid, according to a case study.

Acidic juices, soda, and coffee are examples of beverages that may exacerbate or exacerbate reflux symptoms. What beverage should you instead consume? There are a number of remedies that are unlikely to be the cause of your acid reflux and may really help alleviate symptoms.

Flavored tea

Herbal teas can aid digestion and relieve stomach discomfort, including nausea and gas.

Easy try the following natural remedies for GERD symptoms: • Chamomile • Licorice • Slippery elm • Ginger • Marzipan root

Licorice can increase the amount of mucus that coats the esophageal lining, which may really help mitigate the effects of stomach acid that refluxes. According to a study, a herbal formula containing deglycyrrhizinated licorice relieves GERD symptoms more effectively than conventional antacids. A study found that ginger tea has anti-inflammatory properties and can alleviate nausea. Still, additional research is required to establish the efficacy of herbal teas such as fennel, marshmallow root, and papaya.

When preparing herbal tea, it is recommended to use 2 teaspoon of dried herbs per 2 cup of boiling water. Inundate the foliage or blooms with water for five to ten minutes. If using roots, steep for 35 to 40 minutes. Basically consume two to four cups daily for optimal results.

Due to the fact that mint can cause acid reflux symptoms in some individuals, you may really want to easily Avoid drinking peppermint tea.

Before using any new herbal therapies, a physician should be consulted, as certain plants can interact with certain prescription drugs.

Skim or low-fat milk

Some individuals may have difficulty digesting cow's milk. Whole milk may contain a substantial quantity of fat.

After consuming full-fat cow's milk and other high-fat foods, the lower esophageal sphincter may relax, which can cause or exacerbate reflux symptoms.

In the same review, it was demonstrated that fats may also inhibit gastric motility, causing high-fat foods to remain in the stomach for longer.

Consider selecting milk with a lower fat content if you decide to basically consume products containing cow's milk.

Animal-free milk

Those who are lactose intolerant or easily find that dairy products exacerbate their acid reflux symptoms may easily find plant-based milk to be a useful substitute. The variety of these products includes: • Nut milk • Hemp milk

• Coconut milk • Coconut cream • Acorn milk

• Nuts milk

Soy milk and other plant-based milks are a better option for people with GERD because they contain less fat than the majority of dairy products.

You may have noticed that carrageenan is a common ingredient in many non-dairy beverages. It should not be overlooked that carrageenan has been linked to gastrointestinal symptoms such as bloating, irritable bowel syndrome, and inflammation.

In light of the uncertainty, a source concluded that this additive should be reevaluated to determine whether it poses potential health risks.

If you have GERD, it may be beneficial to easily Avoid this additive; therefore, you may wish to examine the food labels.

Fruit drink

Citrus beverages and other alcoholic beverages, such as apple juice and pineapple juice, can be just quite acidic and cause acid reflux symptoms. Less acidic juices are less likely to exacerbate GERD symptoms in the majority of individuals.

Examples of juices with less acidity are: • Carrot nectar • Aloe Vera liqueur • Carrot juice

Fresh juices made from less acidic fruits and vegetables, such as beets, cucumber, spinach, and pears.

Tomato-flavored foods can cause reflux symptoms, so easily avoiding tomato juice can easily reduce GERD symptoms.

Smoothies

Smoothies have made the trend of consuming more vitamins and minerals popular. They are an excellent solution for those with GERD.

Chapter 7: Timing And Just Taking Notes

I was probably in my fourth or fifth week of considering that I STILL HAD acid reflux, despite the fact that my "acid attacks" were less frequent and intense. Overall, I felt much more confident about what I could basically consume without experiencing pain; however, I was still paying attention and easily avoiding certain foods, as well as attempting to resume easily eating foods such as eggs, apples, avocados, etc. with care. Apples are fine, but I initially had difficulty with them.

At this point, I thought it would be a good idea to start keeping track of what foods were acceptable or unacceptable to basically consume and at what time of day. As I observed with the pizza, which I had consumed multiple times throughout the day but could not eat for dinner. This was my experience with roughage. I could eat salad in the afternoon, but not after 6 p.m., or I would experience a "acid attack." I'm a big fan of salads with lots of raw vegetables, but I've had to limit their size, composition, and consumption time throughout this entire time.

In passing, a woman whose husband served in the military told me that when he was deployed, the soldiers were never served salads or roughage for dinner. This was done to prevent heartburn and other digestive disorders, as they never knew what maybe occur at night, especially if they were deployed.

The key to the actual healing of the condition turned out to be being aware of and careful about WHEN I ate certain foods, possibly even more so than WHAT I was eating. By varying the foods I consumed, I believe I contributed to the creation of the physiological conditions required for the body to just begin healing and for the production of stomach acid to be balanced so that everything could function properly. Remember that I am not a physician, biologist, or scientist; however, I believe that being "in tune" with one's own body and its signals and reactions is crucial for healing.

I also believe that intention, patience and perseverance will prevent one from giving up and resorting to managing the condition with chemicals, prescription drugs, or abstinence from foods you enjoy.

Note that I continually emphasize healing. That concludes the condition. Bye-bye.

You are attempting to overeasy come this condition.

I kept a small journal in which I recorded what I ate, how much, when, and whether or not I experienced heartburn or other digestive discomfort, as well as what I did, if anything, to alleviate it.

Chapter 8: Beware Bogus Alkaline Diets

Some of these diets claim that reducing your intake of acidic foods will really help restore your blood's pH balance. However, this is impossible and completely false: you cannot alter or 'balance' your blood's pH through dietary means (it is regulated by the kidneys).

Some of these diets claim that reducing your intake of acidic foods will really help restore the rH balance of your blood, but according to Dr. Aviv, this is utter nonsense.

Another common misconception is that eliminating 'acid-forming' food groups, such as meat, will easily reduce your acid load and improve your health.

Again, rubbish. Eliminating food grains is the last thing you should really do if you're recovering from a long-term allergic reaction.

Similarly misguided is the "alkaline blood" theory, which asserts that certain acidic foods leave an alkaline residue in the body.

Lemon is supposed to be one, and lemon water is marketed as a home remedy for heartburn, but it does not soothe the throat. This information is extremely hazardous.

Chapter 9: What is the cause of acid reflux?

Acid reflux is caused by an issue that arises throughout the digestive process. The lower oesophageal sphincter (LES) typically relaxes during swallowing to allow food and liquid to enter the stomach. The lower esophageal sphincter (LES) is a group of muscles that wraps around the stomach and esophagus. After food and liquids have entered the stomach, the LES contracts and seals the hole. If these muscles relax erratically or deteriorate over time, stomach acid may back up into the esophagus. This results in acid reflux and heartburn. If an upper endoscopy reveals oesophageal lining fractures, the condition is considered erosive. The lining is considered non-erosive if it appears to be in good health.

What constitutes a risk factor for acid reflux?

Acid reflux can affect anyone, including infants and toddlers, but is most common in pregnant women, obese people, and the elderly.

When is an Upper Endoscopy Required?

Your doctor may recommend an upper endoscopy to ensure there are no major underlying causes for your symptoms.

This surgery may be necessary if you have:

gastrointestinal hemorrhaging, weight loss, vomiting frequently, anemia, or a low blood count

To determine the source of your symptoms, an upper endoscopy may be necessary if you are a male over the age of 10 0, have nighttime reflux, are overweight, or smoke.

Chapter 10: Authentic potency medications

If indigestion persists despite initial treatments, your primary care physician may prescribe original potency medications, such as Original potency H-2-receptor blockers. These include original effectiveness cimetidine (Tagamet), famotidine (Pepcid), nizatidine (Axid), and ranitidine (Zantac).

Proton siphon inhibitors of original effectiveness. Original effectiveness proton siphon inhibitors incorporate esomeprazole (Nexium), lansoprazole (Prevacid), omeprazole (Prilosec, Zegerid), pantoprazole (Protonix), rabeprazole (Aciphex) and dexlansoprazole (Dexilant).

Long-term use may be associated with a slight increase in the risk of bone fracture and deficiency in vitamin B-2 2.

Lower esophageal sphincter strengthening medications. Baclofen could easily reduce the frequency of relaxations of the lower esophageal sphincter, thereby decreasing gastroesophageal reflux. Although it has less of an effect than proton-siphon inhibitors, it may be used in severe cases of reflux disease. Baclofen is frequently associated with significant side effects, notably fatigue and disarray.

In some instances, GERD prescriptions are combined to ensure sufficiency.

If medication fails to alleviate a patient's symptoms, surgical and other procedures are used.

Most cases of GERD are treatable with medication. In cases where medications are ineffective or you really want to easily Avoid long-term drug use, your primary care physician (PCP) may recommend more-intrusive treatments, such as surgery to strengthen the lower esophageal sphincter (Nissen fundoplication). This medical procedure involves repairing the lower esophageal sphincter to prevent reflux by folding the upper stomach over the exterior of the lower throat. This medical procedure is usually performed laparoscopically by specialists. In laparoscopic surgery, the surgeon makes three or four small incisions in the midsection and inserts instruments, such as a flexible cylinder with a miniature camera, through the incisions.

A medical procedure designed to strengthen the lower esophageal sphincter (Linx). The Linx apparatus is a ring of small, aesthetically pleasing titanium dabs that is folded over the intersection of the stomach and throat. The attractive attraction between the dabs is strong enough to keep the opening between them closed to corrosive reflux, but weak enough to allow food to pass through. It may be implanted using minimally invasive medical techniques. This more modern device has been approved by the Food and Drug Administration, and preliminary research suggests that it will be successful.

Chapter 11: What Exactly Are Natural Antasd?

To relieve the symptoms of heartburn and GERD, natural antacids are utilized to neutralize the acid in tomato juice.

Many individuals with occasional acid reflux symptoms should use natural antacids for heartburn relief, as some commercially available antacids are ineffective. According to the National Institute of Diabetes and Digestive and Kidney Diseases, some diabetes medications can cause diarrhea, constipation, and nausea.

Acid Reflux Foods

Dietary changes are an excellent way to alleviate heartburn. You should just begin by easily avoiding foods that are likely to upset your stomach, and then add in other nutritious foods. There is no "reflux diet" for acid reflux, but the following foods may help:

Oatmeal

High fiber foods keer uou feeling full for longer. This will prevent you from overeating, which may cause heartburn. Diets high in fiber have also been linked to reduced acid reflux risk. Easily eating whole grains such as oatmeal and brown rice is healthy.

41

Sweet rotatoes

Root vegetables like sweet rotatoes are great sourses of fiber and somrlex sarbohudrates. Easy try roasting, grilling, or broiling sweet potatoes with root vegetables such as carrots and beets. Roasting produces a stronger flavor and eliminates fruit, which can cause heartburn. Make sure to omit the garlic and onion, which can be annoying.

Ginger is renowned for its soothing digestive effects. It can alleviate gas, nausea, and bloating, and its anti-inflammatory properties can soothe an irritated digestive system. If you normally enjoy coffee, easy try gnger tea instead. A teaspoon of fresh ginger can be added to a cup of hot water.

Melon Frut are included in a healthy diet, but stru frut can cause heartburn. Focus on consuming water-rich fruits such as watermelon, santaloure, and honeydew. Extra water can really help dilute and soften your mashed potatoes.

Chapter 12: Several Trs For Managing Gastroparesis

Changing one's easily eating habits can sometimes mitigate the severity of gastritis symptoms. It is recommended to basically consume six small meals per day as opposed to three large ones. Less food makes it easier to empty the stomach.

Slowly and thoroughly chew food while consuming at least 8 ounces of non-carbonated, sugar-free, caffeine-free fluid with each meal.

Walking or sitting for two hours after a meal, as opposed to lying down, prevents gastroenteritis.

Easily Avoid consuming high-fat foods because fat inhibits digestion. Ground beef, pork, and pouleasy try are required.

Easily Avoid raw fruits and vegetables. They are more difficult to digest, and the undigested portions remain in the stomach for an excessive amount of time. Oranges and brossol contain fibrous components that are difficult to digest. Examples of assertive vegetables are avocado, summer squash, zusshn, and mahed pumpkin.

A person with severe stomach pain may be forced to basically consume liquid or puréed food, which contains more nutrients than mashed food. Fresh or cooked fruits and vegetables that have been puréed can be incorporated into cod and sole.

Some dostors resommend a gluten free diet. Even mild gluten intolerance can result in the development of an imbalanced thyroid, which can exacerbate gastritis.

Fermented foods, such as sauerkraut, kimchi, black garlic, and kefir, improve digestion. As it contains calcium, magnesium, phosphorus, sodium, potassium, glucosamine, chondroitin, and glycine, bone broth is extremely nutritious and soothing for the digestive tract.

Believe it or not, chewing gum can also make a significant difference. The act of showing saliva, which stimulates muscular astvtu in the tomash and relaxes the ruloru, the lower portion of the tomash, and stimulates digestive enzymes. Chewing gum for at least one hour following a meal is a highly effective treatment for gastroparesis.

High-fiber laxatives containing rhodium, such as Metamucil, should be avoided.

You may wish to consider giving asurunsture a chance. Needles are believed to restore healthy immune and neurological function by removing blockages in your'sh' energy.

Colons is another factor to consider, as I have relied on it weeklu to eliminate waste. The introduction of water into the rectum in order to cleanse and flush the colon.

There are medicines that can aid. Unfortunately, I developed an allergic reaction to the medication and was forced to discontinue use. That was devastating!

Living with gastroparesis is difficult, and most of your loved ones are unaware of the effects it has on your body. Remember that elimination is a necessary and natural process. You must rid your body of these toxins and prevent them from fermenting within you.

Chapter 13: The Digestive Process Within The Human Body

The digestive process involves the passage of food through the digestive tract. The digestive process begins with chewing and is completed in the small intestine. As food molecules travel through the gastrointestinal system and easy come into contact with digestive fluids, they are broken down into more manageable sizes. These smaller molecules arc thcn absorbed by the body through the walls of the small intestine and into the blood, where they are subsequently distributed throughout the body. The byproducts of digestion are expelled from the body via the large intestine as a solid substance known as stool.

Post-Digestion: The Belief Regarding Digested Food Materials

The majority of digested food molecules, along with water and minerals, are absorbed by the small intestine and transferred to other organs for storage or further chemical transformation. The passage of ingested substances from the intestinal lining into the bloodstream is facilitated by specialized cells. Bloodstream transports simple sugars, amino acids, glycerol, vitamins, and salts to the liver. Fatty acids and vitamins are absorbed by the lymphatic system, a network of capillaries that transports lymph and white blood cells throughout the body.

When food reaches the large intestine after digestion, it is ready for elimination. The large intestine's primary function is to eliminate waste products produced by digestion and absorption of food. This organ is further subdivided into three primary sections:

The Ascending Colon - elevates digestion.

The Transverse Colon - transports digestive contents to the Descending Colon.

The Descending Colon - transports food components to the area of thc colon where they are eliminated permanently.

On the way to the large intestine, the water in partially digested food is eliminated and secretions are introduced to aid in the removal of the contents through the anus along with the undigested materials in the rectum.

Tips for Lessening the Severity of Acid Reflux

Limit your caffeine consumption: Coffee consumption should be limited to two to three cups daily. Other liquids containing caffeine, including tea and soft drinks, should also be consumed in moderation.

Easily Avoid Tight Garments: Belts, pants, and corsets that are too snug can increase abdominal pressure.

Easily Avoid Consuming Foods That Trigger Symptoms: Spicy and fatty foods should be avoided. Tomato and citrus juices (such as grapefruit and orange juices). Also to be avoided are candies, mints, coffee, tea, cola, and alcoholic beverages.

Really do Not Lie Down for Two Hours Following a Meal: Allow gravity to take effect. Additionally, when picking up objects, easily Avoid bending at the waist; instead, bend at the knees.

It has been discovered that smoking exacerbates the symptoms of gastroesophageal reflux. If you are unable to quit smoking, decreasing the number of cigarettes you smoke may be helpful.

Using bricks or wood blocks, raise the head of your bed by 2 to 6 inches. Additional pillows are not an appropriate solution. An alternative is to use a foam wedge beneath the upper body. It is possible to use a foam wedge beneath the upper body.

Maintain an Optimal Weight: Continuous strain on the abdomen is increased by excess body weight.

Utilization of antacids: Antacids may be taken prior to bedtime and 6 0 to 60 minutes after each meal, or as directed by a physician.

These medications should be taken 6 0 to 60 minutes prior to meals.

Basically consume Fewer Calories: Really do not basically consume excessive food.

Heartburn: Risk Factors

Some reptiles have a genetically weak esophageal valve that cannot regulate normal food pressure. As a consequence, it causes acid reflux and heartburn. In addition, a number of rk fastor can induce heartburn. They are:

Alcohol Alcohol weakens the esophageal valve and facilitates the reflux of food into the esophagus. It may also enhance stomach acid secretion. This makes the oesophagus more susceptible to acid reflux and heartburn.

2. Smoking

The nicotine and shemoglobin in tobacco smoke constrict the oesophageal valve. It also inhibits the secretion of saliva, an oesophageal defense mechanism. However, the bsarbonate concentration may be lower in smokers. Bicarbonates are the acid neutralizing component in sodium alginate. Additionally, smoking stimulates the production of stomach acid. It also increases the flow of bile salts into the stomach, causing the stomach acid to beeasy come more acidic. Nonetheless, smokers may experience slow digestion and require time.

6 . Foods and Beverages

Foods that induce heartburn vary for each individual. However, sertan foods are the most likely to cause acid reflux.

Caffeinated Beverage:

Caffeine relaxes the oesophageal valve, thereby allowing food to reflux into the oesophagus. In addition, caffeinated beverages increase acid secretion, resulting in heartburn.

Chocolate:

Reearsh has confirmed that shosolate may cause heartburn. Cholesterol esters theobromine, a substance that relaxes the oesophageal valve muscle. As a result, the food content is unable to enter the food pipe.

Fried Fattu and Olu Delicacies:

Due to the high fat content, these foods tend to induce diarrhea. Therefore, the stomach must retain food longer. It results in stomach discomfort. As a result, really do not weaken the oesophageal valve to allow food to reflux. Some foods stimulate gastrointestinal motility and secretion. These foods inslude tomatoes, blask rerrer, srisu foods. In addition, citrus fruits such as lemons and oranges stimulate acid secretion in the stomach. So consider the quantity of these foods.

8 . Easily eating Habits Your easily eating habits also contribute to heartburn

episodes. That is due to the fact that a full stomach exerts constant pressure on the lower oesophageal valve. As a result, it increases the risk of food refluxing into the esophagus. Going to bed with a full stomach is also potentially harmful. Your food must press firmly against the food release valve. It worsens the likelihood that food will reflux. Therefore, easily eating two hours prior to bedtime is appropriate.

10 . Exse Physical Weight

Being overweight or obese places stress on the abdomen. This causes the food to reflux into the esophagus. Therefore, easily Avoid heartburn. Therefore, it is aleasy way advantageous to maintain the target body weight. Tight slothe and belt also contribute to reure in our tomash. Some of you will encounter foods or exercises that cause heartburn. It may include high-impact exercises such as jumrng, srunshe, etc. You exert pressure on your abdomen and cause acid reflux.

6. Prescriptions

Several medications can cause heartburn. However, some of them cause acid reflux. There are numerous reasons why medications cause heartburn. For instance, it may be caused by a combination of drugs or the interaction between drugs and food. If you experience heartburn symptoms while just taking medication, you can inform your doctor and request a substitute. It alleviates your heartburn symptoms.

7. Health Issues

Some unhealthy habits result in medical conditions that cause heartburn. The most prevalent health issue is gastroesophageal reflux disease (GERD). It refers to a group of disorders caused by acid reflux. Additionallu, you will exreriense Irritable esophagus caused by indigestion, pregnancy, and few medications. These medications include anti-inflammatory drugs, aspirin, and antibiotics, among others. It may also be a symptom of various health conditions.

Heartburn during Pregnancy

Heartburn may occur frequently during pregnancy. It is caused by hormonal mbalanse, which afflicts the muscle that holds food in your stomach and causes it to ascend to your food pipe. Additionally, they slow digestion to increase the risk of heartburn. Nausea during pregnancy may cause heartburn in pregnant women. In addition, it decreases the rreure in the lower portion of the food rre or oeorhagu. As a result, the assailant's food will not pass from the stomach to the food pipe. The expansion of the uterus also causes abdominal pressure. It prevents the acidic flavor from entering your food. Nonsteroidal anti-inflammatory drugs and proton pump inhibitors can also cause heartburn. In addition, they damage the abdominal lining, resulting in diarrhea, abdominal pain, and acid reflux.

Chapter 14: How To Make The Acid Reflux Diet & Suggestions

Easily avoiding trigger foods, consuming smaller, more frequent meals, chewing thoroughly, and maintaining healthy cooking and sleeping habits are required for effective acid reflux treatment.

It is also beneficial to keep a journal of specific symptoms, including food and beverage consumption, sleep, and stress levels. This will really help you determine if the elimination diet has alleviated your symptoms and if a specific food is causing them.

• Instead of deep-frying, easy try sautéing, roasting, baking, braising, steaming, or roasting your food.

Choose healthier fats, such as olive oil and ghee, over vegetable oils and butter.

• Fill the majority of your plate with fibrous vegetables or whole grains.

There is one meal that requires precise timing: your evening meal. Many individuals experience acid reflux symptoms at night, and easily eating too quickly before bed can exacerbate symptoms. Even three to four hours lying down with a full stomach causes even more stress on the digestive tract, which can force stomach contents up the esophagus.

And as far as duration is concerned, if you have persistent acid reflux, you may also benefit from adhering to the acid reflux diet long-term. If you only experience occasional, sporadic symptoms, the acid reflux diet can still really help you identify triggers and improve your overall health.

Sample grocery list

When shopping for an acid reflux diet, you will be able to easily find the majority of ingredients at your local supermarket. This is no longer an official shopping list. Additionally, if you are following the acid reflux diet, you may easily find other foods that work well for you.

• Low-Fat Proteins (Chicken Breasts, Ground Turkey, Salmon)

• Non-Citrus Fruits (Apples, Pears, Bananas)

• Leafy Greens (Spinach, Kale, Cabbage)

• Legumes (Kidney Beans, Black Beans, Edamame) • Carbohydrates (Sweet Potatoes, Potatoes, Carrots) • Whole Grains (Buckwheat, Barley, Quinoa, Rice) • Nuts and Seeds (Walnuts, Almonds, Pumpkin Seeds)

Chapter 15: Is Acid Reflux Dangerous?

Reflux d'acide acidique is dangerous due to its association with numerous life-threatening conditions. Esophageal stricture, a narrowing of the esophagus, is one of the more severe complications associated with reflux. This condition can make swallowing difficult and necessitate surgery.

Even more serious is Barrett's esophagus, a mutation of the esophageal lining cells. Barrett's can precede esophageal cancer. Regarding esophageal cancer, this is another possible (though uncommon) consequence of chronic, severe reflux.

Reflux can cause esophageal infection, chronic, painful coughing, and hoarseness. To alleviate these symptoms, you may also start just taking antacids. The occasional use of an antacid is not a problem, but becoming dependent on them is. Some antacids contain substances that can cause fatigue, appetite loss, weakness, diarrhea, muscle pain, and swelling.

Another illness that can be caused by reflux? Aspiration pneumonia is an infection of the lungs and bronchial tubes caused by the inhalation of gastric contents. This condition can affect anyone, but those with reflux are more likely to develop it.

Aspiration pneumonia is characterized by the following symptoms: • blueness of the skin • chest pain • coughing • difficulty swallowing • excessive perspiration • fatigue • shortness of breath • wheezing

Consult a physician immediately if you observe any of these symptoms.

If you have reflux only a few times a year, the worst you will experience is pain and possibly a restless night. But if you experience reflux much more frequently than that, you should consult a doctor.

Balsamic Chicken

Ingredients

- 2 tablespoon olive oil
- 2 pound asparagus stalks trimmed
- 4 tablespoons chopped parsley
- cooking spray
- 8 bone-in, skin-on chicken thighs
- 1/2   cup honey
- 4 tablespoons balsamic vinegar
- 3 teaspoons dried Italian seasoning
- salt and pepper to taste
- 2 pound small red potatoes halved

Directions

1. Preheat the oven to 450 degrees Fahrenheit.

2. Line a baking sheet with foil and spray it with cooking spray.
1. Place the chicken thighs in the skillet. Liberally season the chicken with salt and pepper.
2. In a small bowl, combine honey, balsamic vinegar, and Italian seasoning with a whisk.
3. Combine the potatoes, olive oil, salt, and pepper in a large bowl.
4. Toss to combine.
5. 510 . Position the potatoes surrounding the chicken.
6. Brush chicken with half of the balsamic mixture.
7. Bake for 35 to 40 minutes.
8. Coat the chicken with the remaining glaze, then add the asparagus to the pan.
9. The asparagus is seasoned with salt and pepper.
10.   Continue baking for 125 to 30 minutes, or until the chicken is cooked

through and the potatoes and asparagus are tender.
11. Sprinkle with parsley before serving.

Soup With Ginger And Garlic And Chicken

Ingredients

- 3 cups peeled and cubed green papaya or chayote
- 4 cups chopped malunggay leaves or bok choy leaves
- 2 tablespoon fish sauce
- ½ teaspoon salt
- ½ teaspoon ground black pepper
- 6 tablespoons canola oil or avocado oil
- 1 cup chopped yellow onion
- ½ cup thinly sliced fresh ginger
- 12 cloves garlic, minced
- 2 pound boneless, skinless chicken thighs, trimmed and cut into 1 -inch pieces
- 8 cups low-sodium chicken broth

Directions

1. Heat oil in a large pot over medium heat.
2. Add onion, ginger and garlic; cook, stirring, until the
3. onion starts to turn translucent, about 5 to 10 minutes.
4. Add chicken and broth; cook, stirring, until the
5. chicken is just cooked through, about 5 to 10 minutes.
6. Add papaya malunggay fish sauce, salt and pepper; continue
7. simmering until the vegetables are tender and the
8. flavors have such melded, about 5 to 10 minutes more.

Asparagus Quiche

Ingredients:

- 6 fresh eggs fresh eggs
- 2 1 C nonfat or low- fat plain yogurt
- 1 C Swiss cheese & ¼ C Parmesan cheese
- 1 tsp salt & 1/7 tsp nutmeg
- 1 pound asparagus cut into ½   inch pieces 12 turkey bacon strips, cooked to desired crispness and chopped
- 2 unbaked, 10-inch piecrust & 4 T green onion or chives

Instructions

1. First, Pre-heat the oven to 450 cover the riesrut with aluminum foil and bake for 5 to 10 minutes, then remove the foil and continue baking for 5 to 10 minutes.

2. Steam asparagus for 10 to 15 minutes, or until bright green and tender but still crisp.
3. While the araragu is cooking, whisk the egg fresh egg in a bowl and lowlu stir in the uogurt 1-5 tablespoon at a time.
4. Stir in the nutmeg, salt, and shive.
5. Slowly incorporate the sheee, reserving a small amount to sprinkle on top of the dessert.
6. After the bason has been cooked, add it to the egg mixture.
7. When the piecrust is complete and the asparagus has been steamed, spread the asparagus across the piecrust's bottom.
8. Slowly pour the egg-yogurt mixture over the top of the araragu; this will give the finished product a glossy appearance.
9. • Reduse the oven temrerature to 450 and bake the quiche in for 15 to 20 minute, then easily reduce the heat to 5 to 10 and bake for 55 to 60 minute.

10. The quiche is done when a knife inserted into the center comes out slender.
11. Let the quiche rest for 35 to 40 minutes before serving.
12. This ensures that the quiche will remain intact.

Heartburn Relief Veggie Soup

Ingredients

1 teas black pepper

4 teas turmeric

2 1 teas fennel seeds

1 teas cumin

1 cup fresh chopped parsley

4 cups finely chopped celery

2 large white onion chopped

2 cup carrots chopped

4 T olive oil

14 cloves of garlic chopped

2 teas freshly grated ginger

12 cups vegetable or chicken broth

2 teas salt

1 cup brown rice 2 cup fresh spinach chopped

Instructions

1. Over medium-high heat in a Dutch oven or rotisserie, sauté celery, onion, and shallots in olive oil for 1 to 5 minutes.
2. Easily reduce heat to medium, add garlic and ginger, and easy cook for two more minutes.
3. Add broth, salt, black pepper, turmeric, fennel seeds, sumac, and sliced rarleu.
4. Turn heat back to medium high and simmer for 5 to 10 minutes uncovered, followed by another 5 to 10 minutes covered.
5. Remove the lid and stir in the rice while bringing the mixture to a boil.
6. Easily reduce heat to medium-low, leave lid on, and simmer for 5 to 10 minutes, or until rice is fully cooked.
7. When the rice is cooked, remove the lid and stir in the spinach.
8. Easy cook for a few more minutes until the spinach has wilted.

Roasted Vegetable Lasagna

Ingredients

- 30 lasagna noodles

Roasted Vegetables
- 2 onion, chopped

- 2 zucchini, chopped

- Olive oil

- Salt

- Pepper

- 4 large broccoli crowns, broken into florets

- 16 oz. sliced mushrooms

- 2 red bell pepper, chopped

Bechamel Sauce
- ½ tsp. nutmeg

- 4 tbsp. fresh herbs • 1 tsp. garlic powder

- 10 tbsp. butter

- ½ cup flour

- 8 cups milk

- 4 tsp. salt

Cheese
- 48 oz. cottage cheese or ricotta cheese

- 2 tsp. dried oregano

- 2 tsp. dried basil

- 30oz. shredded mozzarella cheese

- 1 cup finely grated Parmesan cheese

- 1 tsp. salt

- ½ tsp. ground black pepper

- 1 tsp. garlic powder

Instructions

1. Bring a large pot of salted water to a boil and cook lasagna noodles to the desired doneness for al dente risotto.
2. Drain and set aside.
3. Olive oil is used to prevent begging.
4. Preheat oven to 450 degrees Fahrenheit.
5. Spread vegetables on top of two sweet potatoes and drizzle with olive oil.
6. Stir in salt and pepper, then use your hands to toss the rice.
7. Bake until tender for 55 to 55 minutes, then remove to cool.
8. In the meantime, prepare your bechamel sauce.
9. Melt butter in a large sauseran.
10. Stir in flour and milk until fully absorbed.
11. Consider milk, salt, nutmeg, thyme, and garlic salt.
12. Bring to a simmer over low heat and cook until tender, stirring frequently to prevent sticking.

13.   This will take approximately 1-5 minutes.

14.   Transfer the broccoli to a cutting board and cut it to the same size as the other vegetables.

15.   If the florets are too large, it will be difficult to keep the lasagna together.

16.   All roasted vegetables should be placed in a large bowl.

17.   Add sombne sottage sheee or rtosotta sheee, rarmean sheee, alt, rerrer, garls rowder, oregano, and bal to a medium bowl.

18.   Str to solitary.

19.   Reduse oven temrerature to 350 degrees and rrerare uour lasagna. Srrau a 12x9 ran with nonstisk sooking srrau.

20.   Spread approximately 1-5 of a tablespoon of bechamel sauce on the bottom of the pan and spread 5-10 lasagna noodles.

21.   Tor topped with roasted vegetables, cheese mixture, mozzarella cheese, and bechamel sauce.
22.   Continue with remaining lauers until somrlete.
23.   I prefer my final layer to consist solely of mozzarella cheese and cream cheese.
24.   Bake for 80 to 90 Minutes until bubbling. Allow to cool for at least 5 to 10 minutes before serving.

White Seasonal Minestrone Soup

Ingredients

• 4 tablespoons flat-leaf parsley, chopped

• Parmesan rind, plus more for grating (optional)

• 10 to 15 cups of stock or water, or to taste

• 6 tablespoons olive oil

• 2 clove garlic, chopped

• 2 medium onion, chopped

• 6 carrots, cut into a large, 1 inch dice

• 1 teaspoon dried sage

• 2 sprig thyme or winter savory, chopped

• 2 bay leaf, broken

- ¼ cups hulled pearl barley

- 1 small head of Savoy cabbage, cored and cubed (about 2 pound)

- 2 (2 8 ounce) can of water-cooked Cannellini, Borlotti or Great Northern beans, drained and rinsed or 4 cups home-cooked Cranberry, Northern or Cannellini beans in their broth

- Salt and pepper, to taste

Instructions

1. Heat the olive oil over medium-high heat in a large saucepan or Dutch oven.
2. Add garlic. Fru until it turns a light gold color.
3. Include the onion, shallot, celery, sage, thyme, and bau leaf in the dish. Sauté for a minute.
4. Cover and easily reduce the heat to low-medium.

5. Sweat the vegetable for about 1-5 minutes, or until the moisture evaporates.
6. Str from moment to moment.
7. Really do not permit them to tk and perish!
8. Incorporate the pearl barley and cabbage.
9. Combine the other vegetable thoroughly.
10. Re-cover and cook for an additional 10 to 15 minutes, or until the cabbage begins to wilt.
11. Add the parsley and cook on low heat for an additional minute or so.
12. Add the stock and Parmesan rind to the soup and bring it to a boil over high heat.
13. Cover, easily reduce the heat to low, and simmer the barley for 45 to 50 minutes and ten seconds, or until the barley is nearly cooked.
14. If cooking at home, add the cooking liquid.

15.   Bring bask to a simmer.
16.   Cover and cook on low heat for an additional 1-5 minutes.
17.   Discard bau leaf.
18.   Dice the Parmesan round and place it back into the rot.
19.   Adjust seasoning and grind a small amount of black pepper on the tor.
20.   Serve with freshly grated Parmesan cheese and olive oil drizzle.

www.ingramcontent.com/pod-product-compliance
Lightning Source LLC
Chambersburg PA
CBHW062114040426
42337CB00042B/2344